HASHIMOTO DIET COOKBOOK

Healing Recipes For Thyroid Health, Inflammation Reduction, And Balanced Hormones

DR ELIAN GRIFFIN

Copyright © [Elian Griffin] [2024]. All rights reserved.

Without the publisher's prior written consent, no portion of this publication may be copied, distributed, or transmitted in any way, including by photocopying, recording, or other mechanical or electronic means, with the exception of brief quotations used in all critical reviews.

DISCLAIMER

The nutritional recommendations and recipes in this book are meant solely for informative reasons. They are not meant to replace the counsel, diagnosis, or care of a qualified medical expert. If you have any doubts about a medical condition or dietary requirements, you should always see your physician or another trained healthcare expert.

All reasonable efforts have been taken by the author and publisher to ensure that the information contained in this book is correct as of the date of publication. Recommendations may alter, though, as medical knowledge is always changing. When using any of the recipes or instructions found here, the user assumes all liability and assumes no risk, whether personal or otherwise. People who have certain dietary requirements or medical issues should speak with a healthcare provider for personalized guidance. The given recipes are only ideas; you may need to adjust them to suit your own nutritional needs, tastes, and tolerances.

When you use this book, you agree to release the publisher, the author, and their representatives from any liability for any claims, damages, liabilities, costs, or expenditures resulting from your use of the book.

TABLE OF CONTENTS

ABOUT THE BOOK

The "Hashimoto Diet Cookbook" is a priceless tool for anyone navigating the symptoms of Hashimoto's disease, an autoimmune thyroid gland disease. It is important to understand how diet affects the disease and how to manage symptoms while also promoting overall health. This cookbook discusses the critical relationship between diet and Hashimoto's, highlighting the importance of nutrient-rich foods in maintaining thyroid health and effectively managing symptoms.

The book gives readers a clear understanding of the fundamentals of the Hashimoto diet approach, enabling them to create meals that support thyroid function and improve nutritional balance. It also teaches readers what foods to avoid and what to include in their diets, enabling them to make well-informed decisions about what to eat based on their individual health needs. Finally, the book emphasizes the importance of diet consistency, showing how small, sustainable changes over time can have a big impact.

This cookbook's foundation is its practical meal-planning strategies, which provide efficient methods for arranging meals to satisfy a range of dietary requirements. It also includes sample meal plans that accommodate different tastes and dietary needs, making the Hashimoto diet accessible and simple to follow. Additional helpful tips for grocery shopping and batch cooking make meal preparation even more efficient, reducing the amount of time required for people with busy schedules.

Specifically created to be tasty and nutrient-dense, the cookbook offers a wide range of breakfast options, including smoothies, breakfast bowls, and gluten-free options. Lunch and dinner recipes accommodate a range of tastes and dietary requirements, from filling salads and hearty soups to protein-rich main dishes and international flavors.

The book emphasizes customization, encouraging readers to modify recipes to fit their specific needs and preferences.

It recognizes the significance of snacks in maintaining energy levels and satiety and offers nutrient-dense snack ideas, homemade energy bars, and guilt-free sweet treats that are suitable for various dietary restrictions, including gluten-free, dairy-free, vegan, and low-carb options.

The cookbook addresses common issues with weight management, food sensitivities, and symptom management with useful advice and solutions, enabling readers to make decisions that support their health journey. It also shares essential cooking techniques and tips to maximize nutrition and flavor, ensuring that meals are not only health-supportive but also enjoyable to prepare.

Through its thorough coverage of Hashimoto's disease, dietary influences, meal planning techniques, and a variety of recipes, the "Hashimoto Diet Cookbook" provides readers with the knowledge and resources they need to take control of their health through diet. I

CHAPTER ONE

HASHIMOTO DIET INTRODUCTION

OVERVIEW OF THE HASHIMOTO'S DISEASE

An autoimmune disorder that affects the thyroid gland, Hashimoto's disease, also called Hashimoto's thyroiditis, is characterized by an immune system that attacks the thyroid inadvertently, causing inflammation and possible damage over time. This can lead to hypothyroidism, or an underactive thyroid, in which the thyroid gland produces an inadequate amount of hormones necessary for metabolism and general health.

Hashimoto's disease can cause a wide range of symptoms, such as weight gain, fatigue, sensitivity to colds, hair loss, and joint pain. To effectively manage their condition, people with Hashimoto's disease must work closely with healthcare professionals. This often entails monitoring thyroid hormone levels and making necessary treatment adjustments to prevent complications and alleviate symptoms.

In addition to taking medication to replace thyroid hormones, diet, and lifestyle changes can be very helpful in managing symptoms and enhancing the overall quality of life for people with Hashimoto's disease. People with the disease must understand the effects of food choices to maximize their health and quality of life.

RECOGNIZING HOW DIET AFFECTS HASHIMOTO'S

Because diet affects inflammation, immunological response, and hormone balance, it is important to manage Hashimoto's disease. Some foods can worsen thyroid dysfunction and inflammation, while other foods can promote thyroid health and general well-being. For example, dairy and gluten are common triggers for inflammation in people with autoimmune conditions like Hashimoto's, so many find relief by reducing or eliminating these foods from their diet.

Alternatively, a diet high in nutrient-dense foods, such as fruits, vegetables, lean proteins, and healthy fats like those found in avocados and nuts, can help support thyroid function and overall health, which can improve symptom management. These foods are also rich in vitamins, minerals, and antioxidants, which can support immune function and reduce inflammation.

In people with Hashimoto's disease, maintaining stable energy levels and supporting metabolic function also requires balancing macronutrients (carbs, proteins, and fats).

A well-rounded diet emphasizing whole, unprocessed foods and limiting refined sugars and unhealthy fats can help improve health outcomes and quality of life for those managing Hashimoto's disease.

THE VALUE OF A WELL-DESIGNED DIET PLAN

To effectively manage symptoms and support overall health, people with Hashimoto's disease must develop a well-structured diet plan. A structured approach ensures that nutritional needs are met while avoiding foods that may exacerbate inflammation or thyroid dysfunction. Meal planning and preparation should be done with thoughtfulness to incorporate nutrient-dense foods that support thyroid function and lower the reactivity of the immune system.

In addition to avoiding or reducing potential trigger foods like gluten, dairy, and processed sugars, a balanced diet plan for Hashimoto's disease usually consists of a variety of whole foods like fruits, vegetables, whole grains, lean proteins, and healthy fats. Meal planning with plenty of vitamins and minerals can also help support immune function and reduce inflammation, two important aspects of managing autoimmune conditions like Hashimoto's.

Personalized guidance and support in developing a diet plan that meets individual needs and preferences while managing Hashimoto's disease can be obtained by working with a registered dietitian or healthcare provider. In addition to meal planning, it's important to take into account factors like hydration, portion sizes, and timing of meals to optimize digestion and nutrient absorption.

To support people with Hashimoto's disease, this cookbook has been carefully crafted to include ingredients that support thyroid health and reduce inflammation, while still being delicious and enjoyable to eat. Each recipe is full of nutritious, delicious food that adheres to the anti-inflammatory diet principles.

This cookbook provides a wide range of simple-to-make breakfasts, lunches, dinners, and snacks that can be incorporated into a well-balanced Hashimoto's diet plan. From nutrient-dense smoothies to filling salads and cozy soups, every recipe is made to support general health and well-being.

Together with recipes, the cookbook offers helpful advice on meal planning, ingredient substitutions, and overcoming dietary obstacles unique to Hashimoto's disease. Its goal is to provide people with the information and tools they need to make well-informed dietary decisions that promote their health and effectively manage their condition.

Starting with small, manageable changes can help beginners starting on a Hashimoto's-friendly diet better manage their symptoms and improve their overall health. Learn about foods that support thyroid health and those that may exacerbate symptoms, like processed foods, refined sugars, and excess caffeine.

Making the shift to a whole foods-based diet with an emphasis on fruits, vegetables, lean proteins, and healthy fats is a good place to start. Try some gluten-free grains like brown rice or quinoa, and if dairy aggravates your symptoms, look into other dairy options like almond or oat milk.

Meal planning and preparation are essential to sustaining diet consistency and preventing temptation or reverting to less healthful options. To save time during busy times, think about prepping meals in bulk. If you need further advice or encouragement, don't be afraid to reach out to healthcare providers or online groups that specialize in managing Hashimoto's disease.

CHAPTER TWO

KNOWLEDGE ABOUT HASHIMOTO'S DISEASE

SYNOPSIS OF HASHIMOTO'S ILLNESS

Diagnosing Hashimoto's disease, also called Hashimoto's thyroiditis, involves blood tests to check thyroid hormone levels and antibodies. Hashimoto's disease is a common, especially among women, autoimmune condition where the immune system attacks the thyroid gland, causing inflammation and potentially leading to hypothyroidism. Symptoms may include fatigue, weight gain, sensitivity to cold, and hair loss.

Effective management of Hashimoto's disease usually entails taking medication to replace thyroid hormones and modifying lifestyle habits, such as diet.

Patients must collaborate closely with healthcare providers to monitor thyroid function and make necessary treatment adjustments.

Knowledge of the autoimmune basis of Hashimoto's disease is critical for making well-informed decisions about managing health.

HOW NUTRITION AFFECTS HASHIMOTO'S

An anti-inflammatory diet rich in nutrient-dense whole foods, such as fruits, vegetables, lean proteins, and healthy fats, can help alleviate symptoms and support overall health.

Many individuals with Hashimoto's find that certain foods, such as gluten, dairy, and processed foods, can exacerbate symptoms. Dietary management of Hashimoto's disease is largely dependent on reducing inflammation and supporting thyroid function.

Before making significant dietary changes, it's important to speak with a healthcare provider or a registered dietitian to ensure individualized recommendations and proper nutrient balance. Some people with Hashimoto's may benefit from following specific diets like the autoimmune protocol (AIP) or gluten-free diets.

Reducing or eliminating potential trigger foods and incorporating thyroid-supportive nutrients like iodine, selenium, and zinc can be beneficial.

WHY NUTRIENT-RICH FOODS ARE IMPORTANT

For people with Hashimoto's disease, a diet high in nutrients is essential to support thyroid function and overall health. Two important nutrients are selenium, which helps regulate thyroid hormone synthesis and metabolism, and iodine, which is necessary for the production of thyroid hormones. Foods high in these nutrients include eggs, seafood, seaweed, Brazil nuts, and seaweed.

Working with a healthcare provider or dietitian to develop a personalized nutrition plan ensures that dietary changes are both effective and sustainable. Avoiding processed foods, refined sugars, and excessive caffeine can also help manage energy levels and reduce symptoms of fatigue often associated with Hashimoto's disease. A balanced diet that includes a variety of fruits, vegetables, lean proteins, and healthy fats provides essential vitamins and minerals that support immune function and reduce inflammation.

TYPICAL SYMPTOMS AND THEIR SIGNIFICANCE

Although Hashimoto's disease symptoms vary greatly, they frequently include fatigue, weight gain, constipation, dry skin, and hair loss. Symptom management is important for people with Hashimoto's disease because these symptoms can affect daily life and general well-being. Knowing how these symptoms relate to thyroid function can help people recognize when their condition may be affecting their health.

Managing symptoms proactively with medication, lifestyle modifications, and dietary adjustments can improve quality of life and lessen the impact of Hashimoto's on day-to-day functioning. For example, fatigue can be debilitating and may require adjustments in daily activities and sleep patterns. Weight gain, which frequently occurs despite efforts to maintain a healthy diet and exercise routine, can be frustrating and may require dietary modifications tailored to individual needs.

GETTING MEDICAL ADVICE BEFORE MAKING ANY DIETARY CHANGES

To fully understand how particular foods and nutrients may affect your thyroid function and general health, especially if you have Hashimoto's disease, you must speak with a healthcare professional before making any major dietary changes. This professional should be knowledgeable about autoimmune conditions and nutrition. They may also suggest blood tests to measure antibodies and thyroid function, which will provide a baseline for tracking changes.

To ensure that dietary changes are safe, effective, and customized to your unique needs, a registered dietitian or healthcare provider can assist you in creating a personalized nutrition plan that addresses nutrient excesses or deficiencies while also taking into account your health goals.

As you work to manage Hashimoto's disease through diet and lifestyle modifications, regular monitoring and adjustments may be required.

Working together with healthcare providers ensures a comprehensive approach to managing Hashimoto's disease and optimizing overall health outcomes. Individuals with Hashimoto's disease can take proactive steps toward improving their health and well-being by understanding symptom management, focusing on nutrient-rich foods, and seeking professional guidance.

CHAPTER THREE

FUNDAMENTALS OF THE HASHIMOTO DIET METHOD

A key component of this strategy is the elimination of potential triggers like gluten, which may exacerbate autoimmune responses in some people. Instead, the diet emphasizes nutrient-dense whole foods, such as fruits, vegetables, lean proteins, and healthy fats, to provide essential vitamins and minerals that support thyroid function and overall well-being. The Hashimoto Diet is designed to support thyroid health, specifically for those with Hashimoto's thyroiditis, an autoimmune condition affecting the thyroid gland.

The Hashimoto Diet entails learning how specific foods can affect inflammation and thyroid function. It promotes eating foods high in antioxidants and anti-inflammatory qualities, like omega-3 fatty acids, which are found in fish like salmon. These foods assist in controlling autoimmune reactions and lessening the symptoms of Hashimoto's thyroiditis. By emphasizing whole foods and avoiding processed foods and artificial additives, people can improve immune system regulation and possibly alleviate some of the condition's symptoms, improving overall health and vitality.

The Hashimoto Diet emphasizes listening to one's body to identify potential food sensitivities or triggers. By emphasizing nutrient-rich foods and avoiding common allergens or inflammatory triggers, people can effectively support thyroid health and manage their autoimmune condition. However, implementing the diet often involves a gradual transition to new eating habits.

IMPORTANT TENETS AND RECOMMENDATIONS

The main goals of the Hashimoto Diet are to manage autoimmune responses and support thyroid health through dietary choices. It places a strong emphasis on eating whole, unprocessed foods that are naturally high in vitamins, minerals, and antioxidants; these include colorful fruits and vegetables (such as leafy greens, cruciferous vegetables, and colorful fruits), as they provide vital nutrients that support inflammation reduction and immune function.

The Hashimoto Diet is centered around avoiding dairy and gluten because these can worsen autoimmune reactions in people with Hashimoto's thyroiditis. Instead, the diet promotes the consumption of grains that are free of gluten, such as quinoa and brown rice, and substitutes for dairy, like almond milk or coconut yogurt.

These substitutions aid in lowering inflammation and promoting digestive health, which is frequently hampered by autoimmune conditions.

The inclusion of high-quality proteins, such as lean meats, fish, legumes, and nuts, is another important Hashimoto Diet tenet. These protein sources offer essential amino acids required for thyroid hormone production and overall metabolic function. People can stabilize blood sugar levels and sustain energy levels throughout the day by balancing meals with sufficient protein, healthy fats like avocado or olive oil, and complex carbohydrates.

Foods high in antioxidants, like berries, leafy greens, and nuts, help neutralize free radicals and support immune health. Omega-3 fatty acids, found in fatty fish like salmon or flaxseeds, are also beneficial for reducing inflammation and supporting cardiovascular health, which can be compromised in individuals with autoimmune conditions. The Hashimoto Diet suggests including nutrient-dense foods that support thyroid function and reduce inflammation.

On the other hand, foods that can aggravate inflammation or cause autoimmune reactions are discouraged on the Hashimoto Diet. These include grains that contain gluten, such as wheat, barley, and rye, which can cause dysregulation of the immune system and digestive problems in sensitive people. Dairy products, especially those that contain lactose or casein, are also generally avoided because they can aggravate inflammation and cause discomfort in some individuals with Hashimoto's thyroiditis.

The Hashimoto Diet discourages the consumption of processed foods, refined sugars, and artificial additives because they can cause inflammation and have low nutritional value. Instead, whole, unprocessed foods that are high in fiber, vitamins, and minerals are the main focus and provide the necessary vitamins, minerals, and fiber to support thyroid health and immune function in general. People can better manage their autoimmune condition and promote long-term health by following this diet and making informed food choices.

MAKING WELL-COMPOSED MEALS

On the Hashimoto Diet, a balanced meal consists of a variety of nutrient-dense foods that support thyroid function and overall health. For example, a typical meal might consist of a serving of lean protein, like grilled chicken or tofu, along with a generous portion of leafy greens and vibrant vegetables, like broccoli or bell peppers. To promote nutrient absorption, healthy fats, like avocado or olive oil, can be used for salad dressing or cooking.

A balanced meal plan that includes enough protein, healthy fats, and carbohydrates ensures that nutritional needs are met while supporting thyroid health and overall metabolic function. Including gluten-free grains or starchy vegetables like sweet potatoes or quinoa helps provide complex carbohydrates for sustained energy levels throughout the day.

These carbohydrates also help to stabilize blood sugar levels and reduce cravings, which can be beneficial for individuals managing autoimmune conditions like Hashimoto's thyroiditis.

People can design a balanced eating plan that supports their health goals and helps manage symptoms related to Hashimoto's thyroiditis by prepping meals in advance and emphasizing whole, unprocessed foods. Including a range of colors and textures guarantees a diverse nutrient intake, and mindful eating practices promote awareness of hunger and fullness cues, which in turn promote overall wellness and vitality.

THE VALUE OF DIETARY CONSISTENCY

Choosing nutrient-dense foods rich in vitamins, minerals, and antioxidants regularly supports thyroid function and overall metabolic health, which can help alleviate symptoms like fatigue, weight gain, and mood swings associated with Hashimoto's thyroiditis. Following the principles of the diet, which include avoiding inflammatory triggers like gluten and dairy, can help individuals reduce autoimmune responses and promote a balanced immune system.

Establishing healthy eating habits and adhering to a balanced meal routine can help individuals better manage their thyroid health and overall well-being over time. Regular meal planning and preparation can help maintain consistency in the Hashimoto Diet by ensuring that nutritious foods are readily available and easily accessible. This helps in avoiding temptations of processed or unhealthy foods that may exacerbate inflammation or disrupt metabolic function in people with autoimmune conditions.

Furthermore, adherence to a consistent diet promotes digestive health and nutrient absorption—both of which are critical for people with Hashimoto's thyroiditis who may encounter gut-related problems or nutrient deficiencies. People can optimize their dietary practices to support immune function and lessen the influence of autoimmune responses on thyroid health by giving priority to whole, unprocessed foods and avoiding common allergens or inflammatory triggers.

CHAPTER FOUR

MEAL PLANNING STRATEGIES

TECHNIQUES FOR PLANNING MEALS THAT WORK

The secret to successfully managing Hashimoto's diet is to plan your meals so that you always have wholesome meals on hand. To begin, schedule some time each week to plan your meals. Take into account your dietary requirements, preferences, and schedule. Choose foods that are high in nutrients and support thyroid health, like whole grains, lean proteins, and an abundance of fruits and vegetables. Aim for balanced meals that include essential vitamins and minerals.

Make a shopping list based on your meal plan to make sure you have everything you need. Next, make a meal plan that includes breakfast, lunch, dinner, and snacks. Use recipes that are easy to make and emphasize whole, unprocessed ingredients. Organize your plan to include a variety of flavors and textures to keep meals interesting.

Finally, think about batch-cooking staples like grains and proteins to streamline preparation throughout the week.

EXAMPLE MENUS FOR VARIOUS NUTRITIONAL REQUIREMENTS

For those who follow Hashimoto's diet, meal plans that are tailored to individual dietary needs are crucial. For example, if you follow a gluten-free, dairy-free, or vegetarian diet, you should plan meals that meet your needs while still supplying vital nutrients.

A gluten-free meal plan might consist of quinoa salads, roasted vegetables, and grilled chicken, whereas a dairy-free plan might have tofu stir-fries and coconut milk-based curries.

To keep your meals interesting and fulfilling, mix and match flavors and cuisines; plan for snacks and think about nutrient-dense options like nuts, seeds, and fruit; adjust portion sizes according to your caloric needs and level of activity; try new recipes and flavors to avoid mealtime boredom and make sure you're hitting your nutritional targets.

TIPS FOR GROCERY BUYING FOR A HASHIMOTO'S DIET

The secret to sticking to a successful Hashimoto's diet is knowing your way around the grocery store. Start by making a thorough shopping list that takes into account your meal plan and dietary needs. Pay special attention to buying fresh produce, lean proteins, and whole grains. Steer clear of processed foods, artificial ingredients, and added sugars. When possible, choose organic products to minimize your exposure to pesticides and additives.

These pointers will help you make sure your kitchen is stocked with healthy ingredients to support your Hashimoto's diet. Carefully read food labels to identify potential allergens or hidden sources of gluten or dairy. Stock up on pantry staples like beans, nuts, and seeds for convenient meal additions. Consider shopping at farmers' markets or local co-ops for fresh, seasonal produce. Plan your shopping trips to minimize impulse purchases and stick to your budget.

IDEAS FOR BATCH COOKING AND MEAL PREP

Meal prep and batch cooking are useful techniques for streamlining meal preparation in Hashimoto's diet. Begin by selecting recipes that are easily multiplied and made in large amounts. Cook grains, such as brown rice or quinoa, in large quantities to use in salads, soups, and grain bowls throughout the week. Bake lean proteins, like chicken or tofu, and roast vegetables to have on hand for easy meals.

Invest in freezer-safe and microwave-safe storage containers for convenient reheating. Label and date your cooked meals for easy identification. Think ahead and prepare meal components (like chopping veggies or marinating proteins) to speed up cooking on busy workdays. Use slow cookers or instant pots for hands-off cooking that produces delicious dishes. Batch cooking and meal prep can help you save time and make sure you always have wholesome options available.

CHANGING MEALS TO SUIT INDIVIDUAL PREFERENCES

Maintaining enjoyment and adhering to Hashimoto's diet requires that meals be customized to individual preferences. Start by experimenting with flavors, spices, and cooking techniques to create meals that suit your palate. Modify recipes to suit particular dietary restrictions or allergies by changing ingredients or portion sizes.

A balanced and satisfying diet that supports your overall health and well-being can be maintained by customizing your meals. Try exploring different cooking methods like grilling, steaming, or sautéing to enhance flavors without compromising nutrition. Use seasonal produce and herbs to add variety and freshness to your meals. Pay attention to your body's cues and adjust meal sizes or ingredients based on hunger levels and energy needs. Incorporate input from family members or friends to create meals that everyone can enjoy together.

RICH IN NUTRIENT SMOOTHIES AND SHAKES

Smoothies and shakes that are high in nutrients will help your body function better throughout the day. These breakfast options are not only delicious but very simple to make. To start, gather your favorite fruits (bananas, berries, and spinach) and protein-rich ingredients (Greek yogurt or plant-based protein powder). Blend these ingredients with a liquid base (almond milk or coconut water) until they are smooth and creamy. If you want to add even more nutrition, think about adding superfoods (chia seeds, flaxseeds, or a scoop of greens powder).

Smoothies and shakes are very adaptable and can be tailored to your taste and dietary needs. You can make them into a creamy chocolate peanut butter creation or a refreshing tropical blend, for example. They are a quick and easy way to get your fill of important vitamins, minerals, and antioxidants without having to spend a lot of time in the kitchen.

These breakfast options can also be readily modified to fit into specific diets, like vegan, paleo, or low-carb diets.

Smoothies and shakes are a great way to start the day off with a healthy dose of nutrients, sustain your energy levels, and support your general health. Try blending different ingredients to find your favorite flavors and textures. Preparing your smoothie or shake takes only a few minutes each morning, and the result will be a nutritious, filling breakfast that will make the rest of your day go well.

BREAKFAST BOWLS THAT INVIGORATE

Breakfast bowls are an excellent way to start your morning with a full and healthy meal. They usually consist of a base of whole grains, like quinoa or oats, which are high in fiber and provide sustained energy. On top of your grains, you can add different fruits, like sliced bananas, berries, or chunks of mango, for natural sweetness and important vitamins.

You can also add nuts, seeds, or nut butter for extra protein and healthy fats.

A common variation is the acai bowl, which is made by blending frozen acai berries with banana and a small amount of almond milk until smooth. Then, you can transfer the mixture into a bowl and garnish it with fresh fruits, granola, and honey for a tasty and eye-catching breakfast. Alternatively, you can make a savory breakfast bowl that includes cooked quinoa, sautéed greens, avocado slices, and a poached egg for a high-protein smoothie.

Breakfast bowls can be made in a variety of ways to suit individual tastes and dietary requirements. They are simple to put together and can be prepared in advance for a convenient grab-and-go option on hectic mornings. Incorporating breakfast bowls into your daily routine will help you feel fuller longer while also providing your body with the essential nutrients it needs to function at its best all day.

A savory and satisfying breakfast option that's high in protein and nutrients can be achieved with creative egg and vegetable dishes. Try different cooking techniques, such as poached, baked, or scrambled eggs paired with a rainbow of colorful vegetables. For a quick and healthy scramble, sauté spinach, bell peppers, and mushrooms in olive oil until soft, then add beaten eggs and cook until fluffy.

Try making veggie-packed frittatas or omelets with your favorite ingredients, such as tomatoes, onions, and spinach, for a more decadent twist. These dishes can be adapted with cheeses, herbs, and spices to add taste without sacrificing nutrition, and they are adaptable enough to be eaten on their own or as a well-rounded meal with whole-grain toast or fresh fruit on the side.

Eggs are a great source of high-quality protein, and vegetables provide fiber, vitamins, and minerals that are important for overall health. Adding creative egg and vegetable dishes to your breakfast repertoire will add variety and guarantee that you're getting a good balance of essential nutrients. All you need to do is master a few simple cooking techniques to create delicious and nutritious breakfast options that will keep you full and energized all morning long.

BREAKFAST IDEAS WITHOUT GLUTEN

For those who are intolerant to gluten or who are on a gluten-free diet for health-related reasons, there are many tasty and nourishing naturally gluten-free breakfast options available. Start your day with a substantial bowl of naturally gluten-free oats topped with fresh fruit, nuts, and a drizzle of honey or maple syrup for sweetness. Oats are naturally gluten-free, but make sure they are labeled as such to prevent cross-contamination.

You can also enjoy classic breakfast dishes like scrambled eggs with a side of avocado or a veggie-packed omelet without worrying about gluten. Another popular gluten-free option is a smoothie bowl made with dairy-free yogurt or coconut milk blended with frozen fruits and vegetables. Top it with gluten-free granola, seeds, and a sprinkle of coconut flakes for added texture and flavor.

Choosing whole foods and naturally gluten-free ingredients allows you to create satisfying meals that meet your dietary needs and preferences.

Whether you're looking to diversify your breakfast routine or are gluten intolerant, exploring gluten-free breakfast options will help you expand your culinary horizons and support digestive health and overall well-being.

IDEAS FOR QUICK AND SIMPLE BREAKFASTS

Either way, overnight oats are a convenient and satisfying breakfast option that can be eaten cold or heated. Prepared the night before by soaking oats in your preferred milk or yogurt and topping it with fruits, nuts, and seeds, overnight oats are perfect for busy mornings when you need a nutritious meal without spending too much time in the kitchen.

Smoothies made with frozen fruits, greens, and protein powder are also easy to blend and can be taken on the go in a reusable container. Another time-saving option is a breakfast wrap or sandwich made with whole-grain tortillas or gluten-free bread filled with scrambled eggs, avocado slices, and spinach. Add a dash of hot sauce or salsa for extra flavor and enjoy a portable breakfast that fuels you throughout the morning.

Including simple and quick breakfast ideas in your routine guarantees that you will prioritize nutrition without compromising on convenience. These meals can be prepared in advance or put together in a matter of minutes, which makes them perfect for busy mornings. By selecting well-balanced ingredients that offer essential nutrients, fiber, and protein, you prepare yourself for a productive day ahead of time without having to worry about laborious meal preparation.

HEALTHY SALADS AND DRESSINGS FOR SALADS

Choosing colorful, fresh ingredients that offer a range of textures and flavors is the first step in making nutritious salads. Start with a base of vitamin- and mineral-rich leafy greens, such as kale or spinach, and add a variety of colorful vegetables, such as bell peppers, cucumbers, and cherry tomatoes, to improve the salad's appearance and nutritional value. For protein, try adding grilled chicken breast, chickpeas, or quinoa for a filling lunch.

Homemade salad dressings are not only healthier but also more customizable to suit individual tastes. For example, basic vinaigrette consisting of olive oil, balsamic vinegar, Dijon mustard, and honey can enhance the flavor of your salad without adding extra calories.

Alternatively, creamy dressings that are made with Greek yogurt as the basis offer a tangy richness that goes well with leafy greens and crunchy vegetables.

When putting together your salad, combine all of the ingredients in a big bowl, making sure that all of the flavors and textures are evenly distributed. Drizzle a little bit of your preferred dressing over the salad right before serving to preserve its freshness.

You can also add extras like crumbled feta cheese, almonds, or seeds to give it more crunch and flavor. Nutritious salads not only supply you with vital nutrients, but they also make you feel full and energized all day long.

FILLING SOUPS & STEWS

Comforting and nourishing, hearty soups and stews are a great option for any meal, especially in the cooler months. To begin, choose a variety of vegetables to use as the base of your soup or stew, such as carrots, celery, and onions. These vegetables add flavor and vital vitamins and minerals. For protein, you can add lean meats like turkey or chicken breast, or plant-based options like lentils or beans.

Use a lot of herbs and spices to improve the flavor profile of your soup or stew. Spices like paprika, cumin, and turmeric add warmth and complexity, while fresh herbs like thyme, rosemary, and parsley add brightness. Simmer your soup or stew for a long time to let the flavors meld together and create a rich, satisfying broth.

Thick soups and stews are satisfying and adaptable; you can adjust the ingredients to suit your tastes and the availability of ingredients. Serve your soup or stew with whole grain bread or a side salad for a complete meal, and store any leftovers in airtight containers for simple reheating later in the week.

TASTY SANDWICHES AND WRAPS

Convenient and portable lunch options that can be tailored to individual preferences include flavorful wraps and sandwiches. To start, use a whole grain wrap or bread as the base, which adds fiber and keeps you feeling full for longer. Then, fill your wrap or sandwich with a variety of ingredients, such as lean proteins like sliced turkey, grilled chicken, or tofu, and fresh vegetables like lettuce, tomatoes, and avocado for extra crunch and nutrients.

Spreads and condiments like mustard, hummus, or pesto can add flavor and moisture to your wrap or sandwich while also adding a distinct taste that goes well with the other ingredients. If you're vegetarian, roasted vegetables combined with a creamy spread can make a filling and healthy lunch.

Flavorful wraps and sandwiches are versatile and can be enjoyed at home, at work, or on the go. To ensure that every bite of your sandwich or wrap is packed with flavor, layer the ingredients evenly and press down gently to meld the flavors together. You can also choose to serve your sandwich or wrap it with a side of fresh fruit or a small salad to complete the meal.

BUDDHA BOWLS IN BALANCE

A base of whole grains, like quinoa, brown rice, or farro, which provide fiber and essential nutrients, and a variety of cooked and raw vegetables, like roasted sweet potatoes, steamed broccoli, and shredded carrots for color and crunch, make up a healthy and stylish meal option that allows for creative flavor and texture combinations.

Lean meats like grilled chicken or tofu, or plant-based options like chickpeas or edamame, can be added to your Buddha bowl to increase its protein content. To bring everything together and improve its flavor, drizzle your Buddha bowl with a flavorful dressing or sauce like tahini, soy sauce, or homemade vinaigrette.

Buddha bowls are not only satisfying but also nutrient-dense, offering a balanced mix of carbohydrates, protein, and healthy fats in every bite.

To garnish your bowl, think of adding toasted nuts, seeds, or fresh herbs for extra flavor and crunch. Arrange your ingredients in an aesthetically pleasing manner to highlight the vibrant colors and textures.

LUNCH IDEAS FOR WORK OR TRAVEL THAT ARE PORTABLE

Picking foods that are simple to pack and don't need to be heated, like salads in mason jars, bento boxes full of different snacks, or wraps, is a great way to ensure that you always have a healthy meal ready to go. It also helps to choose ingredients that travel well and can survive being kept in a lunch bag or cooler.

Pack items like pre-cut veggies, individual servings of hummus or yogurt, and fresh fruit for a balanced meal. If you want to avoid using vending machine options for energy, think about including healthy snacks like nuts, trail mix, or energy bars in your portable lunch to save time in the morning.

When packing lunches for travel, make sure perishables are kept cool and safe to eat by using insulated containers or thermal bags; steer clear of foods that go bad quickly in warm weather and choose shelf-stable or refrigerated options until ready to eat.

HIGH-PROTEIN MAIN COURSES

For your Hashimoto Diet Cookbook, when it comes to high-protein main dishes, try to include lean sources that are easy to digest and good for thyroid health, like grilled chicken breast marinated in herbs and olive oil and served with quinoa or steamed vegetables; or baked salmon seasoned with lemon and dill and served with a vibrant salad of mixed greens, cherry tomatoes, and avocado. These dishes not only provide essential amino acids but also important nutrients like omega-3 fatty acids and antioxidants.

If you would rather eat plant-based foods, try lentil and vegetable stew cooked with fragrant spices like cumin and turmeric. This dish is high in fiber and plant-based protein, which supports digestive health and gives you long-lasting energy. Alternatively, try this satisfying, high-protein, easy-to-make dish called tofu stir-fried with broccoli and bell peppers. Both of these dishes are great for helping you stay within the Hashimoto Diet guidelines while still maintaining blood sugar balance and supporting overall well-being.

To make your recipes more appealing and varied, try experimenting with lean beef or turkey, tempeh, or beans. By adding a variety of proteins, you'll keep your meals interesting and give your body a wide range of nutrients that are essential for thyroid function and general health.

To maximize energy levels and support a balanced diet specific to Hashimoto's, balance your protein intake with healthy fats and complex carbohydrates.

VEGETABLE-BASED MAIN COURSES

For your Hashimoto Diet Cookbook, you should make vegetable-focused entrees that showcase the tastes and nutritional advantages of different veggies while keeping cooking easy and fun. For example, you could make a roasted vegetable medley, which is a colorful dish that tastes good and is high in vitamins and minerals. It also includes seasonal favorites like carrots, sweet potatoes, and Brussels sprouts tossed in olive oil and seasoned with herbs like thyme and rosemary.

An additional suggestion would be to make a stir-fry with colorful bell peppers, mushrooms, and snap peas sautéed in a light soy sauce and ginger dressing with zucchini noodles.

This dish is low in calories and carbohydrates and provides an abundance of vitamins and antioxidants that are important for thyroid health. Alternatively, you could make stuffed bell peppers, which are a visually appealing and easily customizable dish that is low in calories and carbohydrates. The filling combination would be quinoa, spinach, and tomatoes seasoned with garlic and basil.

Vegetable-based soups, like creamy cauliflower soup or hearty minestrone loaded with beans and leafy greens, can offer satisfying meals that are both nourishing and supportive of thyroid function. When you include a range of vegetables in your recipes, you'll make sure that your diet is nutrient-dense and that the dietary requirements of those who have Hashimoto's disease are met.

ONE-POT DINNERS FOR SIMPLE CLEANING

Starting with recipes like chicken and vegetable stir-fry cooked in a single skillet with sesame oil and tamari sauce, which combines protein, vegetables, and healthy fats in one easy-to-make meal that requires minimal cleanup, or quinoa pilaf with mixed herbs, chickpeas, and diced vegetables simmered in vegetable broth until tender and flavorful, are convenient ways to simplify meal prep and cleanup while following the principles of the Hashimoto Diet.

If you're a seafood lover, try this shrimp and rice paella cooked with bell peppers, peas, and saffron-infused broth. It's a filling dish that also provides lean protein and complex carbohydrates that you need for long-term energy. One-pot meals are a great way to cook quickly without sacrificing flavor or nutritional value—a feature that makes your Hashimoto Diet Cookbook stands out.

One-pot meals are a practical choice for incorporating into a Hashimoto Diet lifestyle because they are versatile and easy to make, whether you're cooking for yourself or your family. Experiment with different combinations of ingredients such as whole grains, lean proteins, and colorful vegetables to create balanced and satisfying meals that support thyroid health.

INTERNATIONAL TASTES AND SKUS

Discovering foreign tastes and variations in your Hashimoto Diet Cookbook offers a plethora of nutrients that are good for thyroid health. To begin, try Mediterranean-style meals, like Greek chicken souvlaki with a side of tabbouleh salad; the combination of lean protein, fresh herbs, and whole grains gives you important nutrients like zinc and selenium, which are vital for thyroid function.

Try making a vegetable stir-fry with tofu and brown rice noodles in a flavorful peanut sauce for a taste of Asia. This dish is high in plant-based protein, fiber, and healthy fats that promote overall well-being and provide sustained energy. Alternatively, try Mexican food with black bean and sweet potato enchiladas topped with avocado slices and homemade salsa verde. Packed with antioxidants and fiber, these enchiladas are a tasty and nutritious choice for eating Hashimoto's-friendly.

International flavors let you sample a range of cuisines while still making sure you get the nutrition you need. Try different herbs, spices, and cooking methods to make tasty, thyroid-healthy dishes.

By embracing international culinary traditions, you'll broaden your horizons and improve your culinary skills while adhering to the Hashimoto Diet's guidelines.

COZY DINNERS SUITABLE FOR ANY TIME OF YEAR

With cozy dinners for every season in your Hashimoto Diet Cookbook, you can be sure that your meals are healthy and suit seasonal produce and tastes. Start with warming stews like this one, which is made with beef and vegetables simmered with root vegetables like potatoes, carrots, and parsnips.

It will keep you warm and supply you with important nutrients like iron and vitamin C.

In warmer months, go for lighter fare like grilled vegetable platters with seasonal favorites like bell peppers, asparagus, and zucchini marinated in olive oil and balsamic vinegar; serve with grilled chicken or fish for a well-balanced meal that highlights the flavors of the season. Another option is a seasonal salad made with mixed greens, fresh berries, nuts, and a light vinaigrette dressing; this dish is refreshing and full of vitamins and antioxidants.

In the spring and fall, try recipes like this one for butternut squash and apple soup with toasted pumpkin seeds; it's full of vitamins A and C, which are good for the immune system and thyroid function. If you make your recipes with seasonal ingredients, you can enjoy delicious, fresh, and nutritionally balanced meals all year long that follow the guidelines of the Hashimoto Diet.

IDEAS FOR NUTRIENT-DENSE SNACKS

Snacks high in nutrients are vital for sustaining energy levels and promoting general health, particularly when following a Hashimoto diet. They should be high in vitamins, minerals, and healthy fats to support optimal thyroid function and help stabilize blood sugar. Raw nuts and seeds are a great source of protein and omega-3 fatty acids; when combined with fruit (bananas, apples, etc.), they add fiber and a naturally sweet taste. Greek yogurt with berries and chia seeds added for extra protein and antioxidants is another excellent option. Vegetables like carrots, cucumbers, and bell peppers dipped in hummus make a crunchy and satiating snack high in vitamins and fiber.

Nutrient-dense snack preparation is easy and can be done ahead of time for convenience. For example, snack packs made with mixed nuts, dried fruits, and a small amount of dark chocolate chips offer a balanced combination of nutrients and sweetness, and spinach, avocado, and almond milk smoothies are a refreshing way to get your fill of vitamins and minerals. These snacks are great for thyroid health, controlling appetite, and warding off unhealthy cravings during the day.

MAKE YOUR ENERGY BARS AND BITS

Making your own energy bars and bites is a great way to avoid buying premade snacks and keep ingredients under control. You can start with a base of oats, nuts, and seeds mixed with natural sweeteners like honey or dates. You can add additional nutrients and flavors by adding coconut flakes, cocoa nibs, or dried fruits. Mix all ingredients, press into a pan, and refrigerate until solid. Cut into bars or roll into bite-sized balls for an easy and portable snack.

Energy bars and bites are great for on-the-go snacking or as a pre-workout boost, providing sustained energy without the crash associated with processed snacks. They are a delicious way to incorporate wholesome ingredients into your Hashimoto diet while satisfying your sweet tooth.

These homemade treats are versatile and can be customized to suit your taste preferences and dietary needs. For example, you can make protein-packed snacking treats that you can eat all day long by rolling the mixture into balls and refrigerating it.

SWEET TREATS WITHOUT GUILT

With a focus on nutrient-dense ingredients and natural sweeteners, such as maple syrup, raw honey, or dates, which provide sweetness in addition to vitamins and minerals, guilt-free sweet treats can be enjoyed on a Hashimoto diet. For instance, ripe avocados can be blended with cocoa powder, maple syrup, and vanilla extract to make chocolate avocado mousse, a creamy dessert that is rich in healthy fats and antioxidants and satisfies chocolate cravings guilt-free.

Frozen banana pops, which are low in added sugars and high in potassium and fiber from bananas, are a refreshing and decadent treat that can be enjoyed guilt-free in moderation. On a Hashimoto diet, enjoying guilt-free sweet treats in moderation can help satisfy cravings while supporting thyroid health and overall well-being.

DELICIOUS SNACKS TO QUENCH YOUR HUNGER

To support energy levels and stabilize blood sugar, choose savory snacks that satisfy cravings and offer a satisfying substitute for sweet treats on a Hashimoto diet. For instance, roasted chickpeas seasoned with olive oil and spices like cumin or paprika make a crunchy, high-fiber, plant-based protein snack that can be eaten on its own or added to salads for extra crunch and flavor.

A delicious addition to your Hashimoto diet plan, these savory snacks are easy to prepare and can be made ahead of time for convenient snacking throughout the week. Another savory option is homemade kale chips, tossed with olive oil and nutritional yeast for a cheesy flavor without dairy; bake until crispy for a nutritious snack that is packed with vitamins A, C, and K. Pairing these savory snacks with a small serving of lean protein like turkey or chicken slices can further enhance satiety and provide a balanced snack option.

SNACK SELECTIONS TO INCREASE ENERGY

Energy-boosting snack options are critical for sustaining focus and stamina throughout the day, especially when following a Hashimoto diet. Select snacks that balance blood sugar levels and prevent energy crashes by combining complex carbohydrates, protein, and healthy fats. For example, apple slices with almond butter provide a healthy balance of carbohydrates, protein, and healthy fats from the nut butter.

Quinoa salad with mixed vegetables and a squeeze of lemon juice and olive oil is another high-nutrient snack. Quinoa is a gluten-free whole grain that offers complex carbohydrates and protein, and vegetables like spinach, bell peppers, and cherry tomatoes add vitamins and minerals. This nutrient-dense snack can be made ahead of time and served cold or at room temperature for a filling and energizing meal.

CHAPTER FIVE

PARTICULAR NUTRITIONAL REQUIREMENTS

OPTIONS FREE OF DAIRY AND GLUTEN

If you're on a Hashimoto diet, it can be very helpful to include dairy-free and gluten-free options. Since gluten, which is present in wheat and related grains, aggravates inflammation and digestive problems in people with Hashimoto's thyroiditis, recipes in this cookbook feature items like gluten-free flours (like almond flour or coconut flour) and dairy substitutes (like almond milk or coconut yogurt). These substitutions not only meet dietary needs but also make sure that meals are easy on the stomach and promote overall health.

Practically speaking, swapping out wheat-based products for gluten-free ones entails using flours derived from nuts, seeds, or grains like quinoa or rice. One can use these flours in baking and cooking to make anything from bread to desserts without sacrificing flavor or texture. Similarly, dairy-free substitutes like nut milk and coconut-based creams offer creamy flavors and textures in dishes that would otherwise be made with dairy. By learning about these swaps and implementing them into regular cooking, people can savor delicious meals while meeting their dietary requirements and supporting their health objectives concerning the management of Hashimoto's thyroiditis.

VEGETARIAN AND VEGAN DISHES

Incorporating vegan or vegetarian variations into a Hashimoto diet can have several advantages, including higher fiber intake, decreased inflammation, and better overall health outcomes. Vegan diets prohibit all animal products, such as meat, dairy, and eggs, whereas vegetarian diets generally exclude meat but allow dairy and eggs.

The recipes in this cookbook accommodate both types of diets by emphasizing plant-based proteins, such as beans, lentils, tofu, and tempeh, which are high in nutrients, such as iron and zinc, which are crucial for thyroid function.

Practically speaking, a vegan or vegetarian Hashimoto diet entails experimenting with various plant-based protein sources and incorporating them into well-known dishes. For example, classic meat-based recipes can be modified by substituting tofu or lentils for protein, retaining flavor and nutritional value. Moreover, adding plenty of fruits, vegetables, whole grains, and healthy fats guarantees a well-balanced diet that promotes general health. Finally, by experimenting with different cooking techniques and flavor combinations, people can find satiating meals that suit their dietary requirements and health goals, promoting long-term adherence to their selected dietary philosophy.

HIGH-FIBRE AND LOW-CARB SUBSTITUTES

On a Hashimoto diet, incorporating low-carb and high-fiber options can help stabilize blood sugar levels, reduce inflammation, and support weight management goals. Low-carb options usually entail minimizing or avoiding refined carbohydrates like white bread, pasta, and sugary snacks; instead, choose lower-carb but high-fiber whole grains, vegetables, and fruits; high-fiber foods like leafy greens, nuts, seeds, and berries promote digestive health and provide essential nutrients without causing blood sugar spikes; recipes in this cookbook center around utilizing these substitutes to support optimal thyroid function and general health.

Putting a low-carb, high-fiber strategy into practice entails swapping out processed carbohydrates for nutrient-dense alternatives. For instance, spiralized zucchini or spaghetti squash can be used in place of traditional pasta, and chia seeds, which are high in fiber, can be added to smoothies or salads to add texture and nutritional value. People can plan meals that balance protein, healthy fats, and complex carbohydrates to make satisfying meals that fit their dietary preferences and health goals for managing Hashimoto's thyroiditis.

RECIPES THAT ARE ALLERGIC-FRIENDLY

To prevent allergic reactions and worsen symptoms, it is essential to develop allergy-friendly recipes for a

Hashimoto diet. Common allergens, such as peanuts, tree nuts, shellfish, and soy, can be avoided or replaced with allergy-friendly alternatives. Recipes in this cookbook emphasize less likely to trigger allergic reactions ingredients, like seeds (like pumpkin or sunflower seeds) in place of nuts, or alternative flours (like cassava or sorghum flour) for those with gluten allergies. By providing allergen-free options, people can feel comfortable preparing meals that meet their dietary requirements and promote their general health and well-being.

In practice, making recipes allergy-friendly means identifying the ingredients that might trigger allergic reactions and choosing safe, nutrient-dense alternatives. For example, substituting peanut butter with sunflower seed butter in recipes guarantees a nut-free option that retains all of the necessary nutrients and flavors. Similarly, in Asian-inspired dishes, tamari or coconut aminos can be used in place of soy sauce to accommodate soy allergies while still preserving the desired flavor profile.

Through awareness of potential allergens and inventive substitutions, people can enjoy a wide variety of tasty, nutritious, and safe meals that support their Hashimoto diet objectives.

To effectively manage Hashimoto's thyroiditis and optimize overall health, personalization of recipes is essential. This cookbook promotes flexibility and creativity in the kitchen, enabling people to customize recipes based on their unique preferences and health objectives.

Whether it's modifying portion sizes to meet nutritional needs, substituting ingredients to accommodate allergies, or adjusting seasoning levels, personalization guarantees that each meal supports individual health needs while promoting enjoyment and satisfaction in eating. People who grasp the concepts of ingredient substitution and portion control can confidently navigate their dietary choices to achieve optimal well-being.

Customization allows for a personalized approach to nutrition, empowering people to make decisions that are in line with their individual health goals. In practice, customizing recipes entails experimenting with different flavors, textures, and cooking methods to suit personal tastes and dietary restrictions. For instance, people may choose to increase protein content by adding extra tofu or beans to a dish, or they may reduce salt intake by using herbs and spices as a seasoning. Portion control can also play a crucial role in managing calorie intake and supporting weight management efforts. By incorporating mindful eating practices and paying attention to their bodies' hunger and fullness cues, people can prepare meals that not only nourish but also contribute to overall health and vitality.

CHAPTER SIX

COOKING METHODS AND ADVICE

CRUCIAL KITCHEN UTENSILS FOR COOKING

When cooking on the Hashimoto Diet, having the right tools in your kitchen can make all the difference. Start with the basics: a good chef's knife for clean, precise cutting; a sturdy, easily cleaned cutting board; a set of stainless steel pots and pans that distribute heat evenly and are long-lasting enough for frequent use; a food processor or blender that works well for smoothies and purees; measuring cups and spoons for precise portioning; and so on.

In addition, think about kitchen tools that make cooking easier, like an instant-read meat thermometer for determining doneness and a vegetable spiralizer for making low-carb pasta substitutes. Moreover, gather multipurpose tools like silicone spatulas and tongs that won't mar non-stick surfaces. Lastly, remember to store leftovers and meal prep in containers that are microwave-safe and stackable for simple organization in your refrigerator or freezer.

HOW TO COOK TO GET THE MOST NUTRITION

Cooking techniques have a big impact on how nutritious your meals are when following the Hashimoto Diet. For example, you can steam vegetables to preserve their vitamins and minerals or lightly sauté them in olive oil to add flavor without sacrificing nutrients.

Lean proteins like fish or chicken can be cooked by poaching them to retain moisture, which makes them soft and easy to digest. Meats can be grilled or broiled to remove excess fat and reduce calories while improving flavor.

Try experimenting with different cooking techniques to find what works best for your taste preferences and dietary needs. Slow cooking is also a great way to prepare hearty stews or soups, as it allows flavors to meld over time and tenderizes tougher cuts of meat.

When possible, incorporate raw foods, like salads or fresh fruit, to maximize enzyme activity and preserve heat-sensitive nutrients.

METHODS FOR ENHANCING FLAVOR

Adding flavor is essential to making delicious meals on the Hashimoto Diet without using a lot of salt or sugar. Try using anti-inflammatory, thyroid-healthy, and aromatic herbs and spices like garlic, ginger, and turmeric to add depth to your dishes.

You can also use vinegar or citrus zest to add brightness and balance flavors. For a savory taste profile, try adding umami-rich ingredients like mushrooms, tomatoes, or nutritional yeast.

If you want to tenderize meat and add flavor, try marinating proteins in yogurt or citrus juice before cooking. Toasting nuts and seeds enhances their crunchiness and brings out their natural oils. Fresh herbs are a great way to add visual appeal and a burst of freshness to dishes.

Carefully layering flavors will help you create satisfying meals that nourish your body and support your dietary goals.

IDEAS FOR LARGE-SCALE COOKING

Whether you're following the Hashimoto Diet and want to make sure you always have wholesome meals available, cooking in bulk can save you time and energy. To start, plan your meals and make a shopping list based on recipes that you can easily scale up. Look for ingredients that can be used in many different ways throughout the week, such as quinoa, beans, or lean proteins. You can also buy large pots or slow cookers to make large quantities of soups, stews, or casseroles that can be frozen for later use.

Make use of time-saving methods such as prepping grains in bulk or roasting veggies, then putting them in separate containers for easy assembly on busy workdays. Label and date your meal preps to monitor freshness and prevent food waste. Include freezer-friendly recipes such as homemade veggie burgers or lasagna that can be frozen for a few weeks and reheated when necessary. By setting aside a few hours each week for meal prep, you'll guarantee that healthy meals are always accessible, even on busy days.

MEAL PRESERVATION AND FREEZING TECHNIQUES

The quality and safety of your meals on the Hashimoto Diet depend on how well you store and freeze them. To prevent freezer burn and preserve flavors, buy airtight containers or freezer bags. Let cooked foods cool completely before packaging to reduce condensation and ice crystals. Label containers with the date and contents for easy identification. Rotate older meals to the front of your freezer for faster consumption.

For optimal thawing and minimal waste, portion meals when freezing into single servings. Soups, sauces, and stews can be frozen flat in resealable bags for effective storage and speedier defrosting. Don't freeze high-water items like lettuce or cucumber because they will become limp and lose their texture when thawed.

To reheat frozen meals, use a microwave or stovetop for uniform heating, adding a little water or broth to keep the meal moist.

Meal preparation on the Hashimoto Diet may be made easy and fulfilling by adhering to these suggestions, which will guarantee that your meals maintain their nutritious content and flavor.

CHAPTER SEVEN

HANDLING HASHIMOTO'S AND WEIGHT MANAGEMENT

Due to the metabolic effects of Hashimoto's thyroiditis, controlling weight can be difficult for those who have the condition. A balanced diet is essential for managing weight; nutrient-dense foods like lean proteins, whole grains, fruits, and vegetables can support metabolic health; avoiding processed foods and excessive sugars helps stabilize blood sugar levels, which aids in weight control; and many people find that weight gain is a common symptom, often linked to hormonal imbalances and reduced thyroid function.

Exercise regularly is equally important because it speeds up metabolism and supports general health. Exercises such as yoga, strength training, or brisk walking can increase energy and help with weight management. You should also check your thyroid hormone levels with your doctor to make sure you are receiving the best possible treatment, which can help you stay in a healthy weight range.

MANAGING INTOLERANCES AND SENSITIVITIES TO FOOD

For people with Hashimoto's disease, food sensitivities and intolerances are common concerns because they can worsen symptoms and impact overall health. One important strategy for managing food sensitivities and intolerances is to identify and eliminate trigger foods, such as gluten, dairy, and soy, which can aggravate thyroid function and inflammation. Keeping a food journal can help monitor responses and spot patterns, which will aid in the elimination process.

Choosing an anti-inflammatory diet high in fruits, vegetables, and healthy fats promotes gut health and lowers the reactivity of the immune system. Trying new grains like quinoa or buckwheat and dairy-free milks like almond or coconut can offer nutrient-dense substitutes without triggering reactions. Consulting a registered dietitian can provide individualized advice in managing food sensitivities and sustaining a balanced diet customized to each person's needs.

KEEPING NUTRIENT NEEDS IN BALANCE

Maintaining optimal thyroid function and immune system health requires balancing nutrient intake, which is critical for managing Hashimoto's and promoting overall health. Iodine-rich foods like seaweed, seafood, and iodized salt, when consumed in moderation, can support thyroid hormone production. Adequate intake of essential nutrients like zinc, selenium, and iodine supports thyroid function and immune system health.

A healthcare provider or dietitian can help determine appropriate supplement dosages based on individual needs and lab results. Zinc, which is abundant in lean meats, legumes, and seeds, aids in thyroid hormone production and immune function. Selenium, which is found in Brazil nuts, fish, and eggs, is essential for reducing thyroid inflammation and supporting antioxidant defenses.

Vitamin D and B12 supplements may also be helpful, as deficiencies are common in individuals with Hashimoto's.

CONTROLLING SYMPTOMS WITH FOOD

Using an anti-inflammatory diet to support thyroid health and lessen autoimmune flare-ups is part of managing symptoms through nutrition. Emphasizing whole, unprocessed foods high in antioxidants and omega-3 fatty acids can help reduce inflammation and support immune function. Leafy greens, berries, fatty fish (like salmon), and olive oil give vital nutrients and enhance general wellbeing.

A gluten-free or dairy-free diet may be beneficial for some people, as these proteins can cause autoimmune responses in susceptible individuals.

Identifying personal triggers and optimizing symptom management can be achieved by experimenting with elimination diets under the supervision of a healthcare professional.

Reducing refined sugars, processed foods, and excessive caffeine can help stabilize energy levels and reduce symptoms like fatigue and mood swings.

LOOKING FOR ASSISTANCE AND RESOURCES

It can be difficult to navigate Hashimoto's disease, but there are resources available to help people manage it well. Participating in online forums or local community networks can offer a wealth of knowledge, a common experience, and emotional support. Making an appointment with a medical team that consists of an endocrinologist, registered dietitian, and mental health specialist guarantees thorough care and individualized treatment plans.

Attending workshops or webinars led by healthcare professionals can deepen understanding and provide practical tools for symptom management. Learning about Hashimoto's and investigating various support avenues can improve quality of life and foster a sense of empowerment in managing this chronic condition.

www.ingramcontent.com/pod-product-compliance
Lightning Source LLC
Chambersburg PA
CBHW061302250726
48653CB00002B/744